Why We Eat Dairy

by Beth Bence Reinke, MS, RD

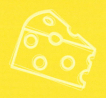
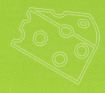
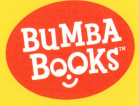
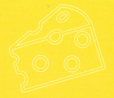

LERNER PUBLICATIONS ◆ MINNEAPOLIS

Note to Educators:

Throughout this book, you'll find critical thinking questions. These can be used to engage young readers in thinking critically about the topic and in using the text and photos to do so.

Copyright © 2019 by Lerner Publishing Group, Inc.

All rights reserved. International copyright secured. No part of this book may be reproduced, stored in a retrieval system, or transmitted in any form or by any means—electronic, mechanical, photocopying, recording, or otherwise—without the prior written permission of Lerner Publishing Group, Inc., except for the inclusion of brief quotations in an acknowledged review.

Lerner Publications Company
A division of Lerner Publishing Group, Inc.
241 First Avenue North
Minneapolis, MN 55401 USA

For reading levels and more information, look up this title at www.lernerbooks.com.

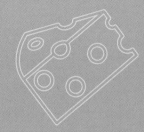

Library of Congress Cataloging-in-Publication Data

Names: Reinke, Beth Bence, author.
Title: Why we eat dairy / Beth Bence Reinke, MS, RD.
Description: Minneapolis : Lerner Publications, [2018] | Series: Bumba books. Nutrition matters | Audience: Ages 4–7. | Audience: K to grade 3. | Includes bibliographical references and index.
Identifiers: LCCN 2017051932 (print) | LCCN 2017057866 (ebook) | ISBN 9781541507678 (eb pdf) | ISBN 9781541503373 (lb : alk. paper) | ISBN 9781541526822 (pb : alk. paper)
Subjects: LCSH: Dairy products in human nutrition—Juvenile literature. | Dairy products—Juvenile literature. | Nutrition—Juvenile literature.
Classification: LCC TX377 (ebook) | LCC TX377 .R45 2018 (print) | DDC 613.2/8—dc23

LC record available at https://lccn.loc.gov/2017051932

Manufactured in the United States of America
1 – CG – 7/15/18

Table of Contents

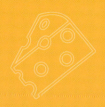

All about Dairy **4**

USDA MyPlate Diagram **22**

Picture Glossary **23**

Read More **24**

Index **24**

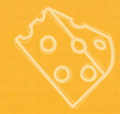

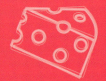

All about Dairy

Dairy foods help make your body strong.

Did you eat dairy today?

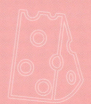

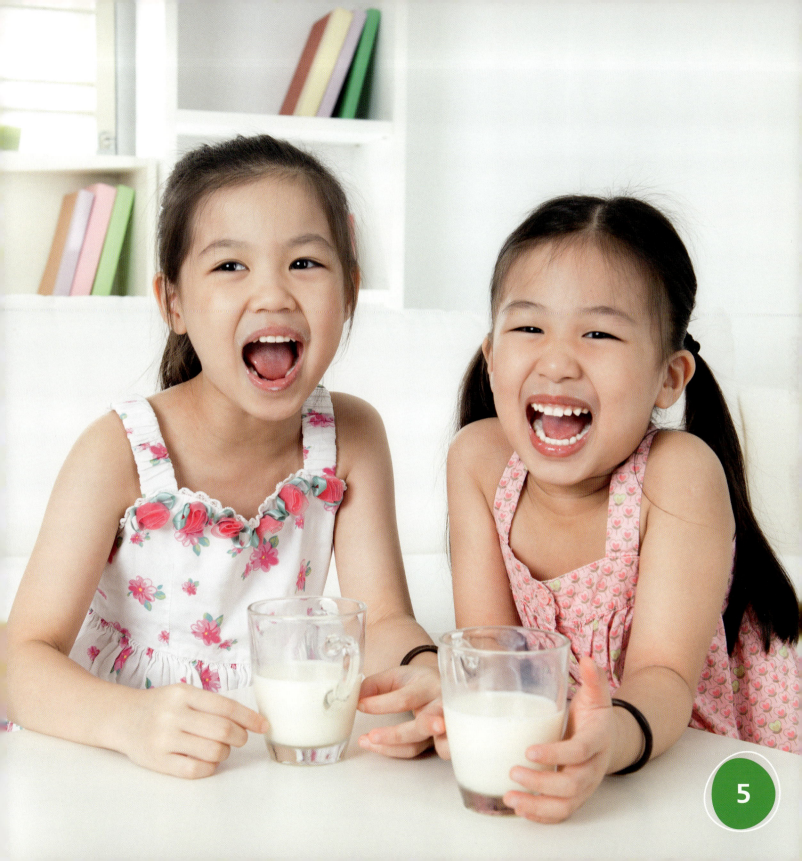

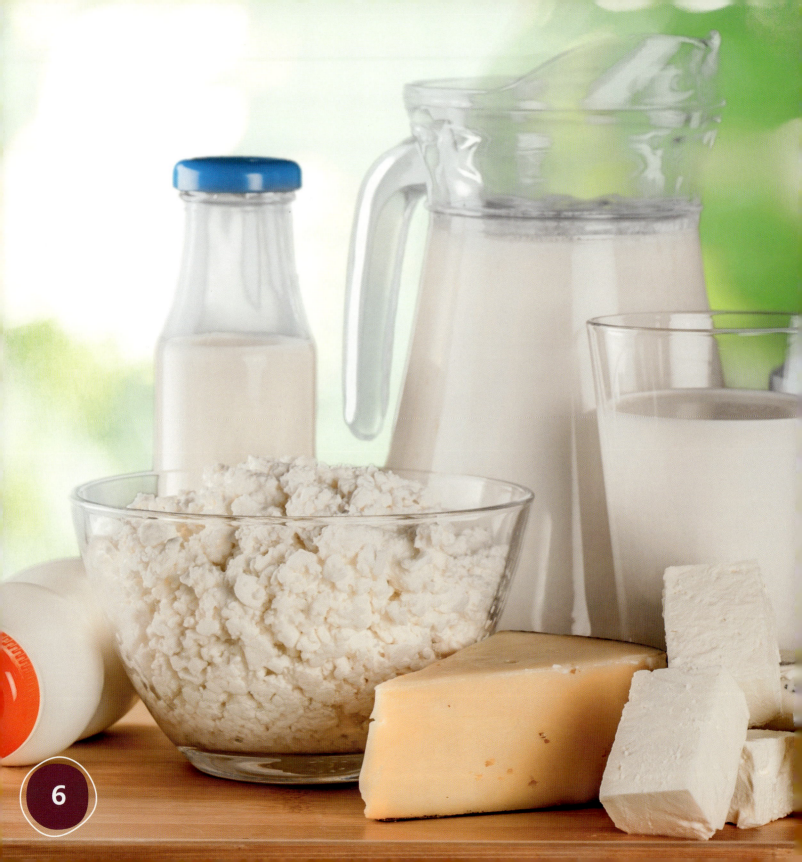

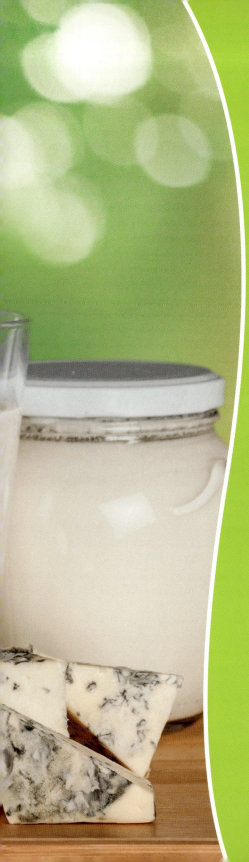
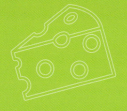

Milk is a dairy food.

So are yogurt and cheese.

They are made from milk.

When do you eat dairy foods?

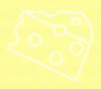

Dairy foods have protein.

Protein helps you grow.

It helps your blood and skin stay healthy.

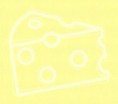

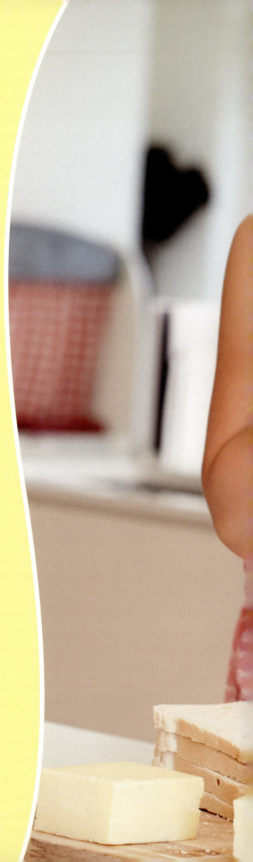

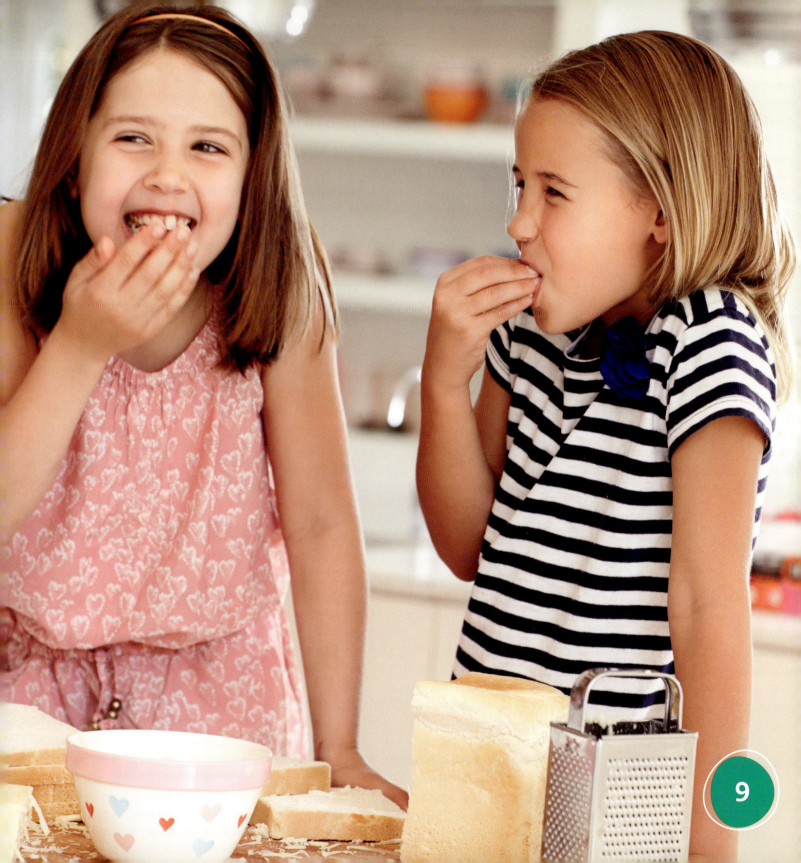

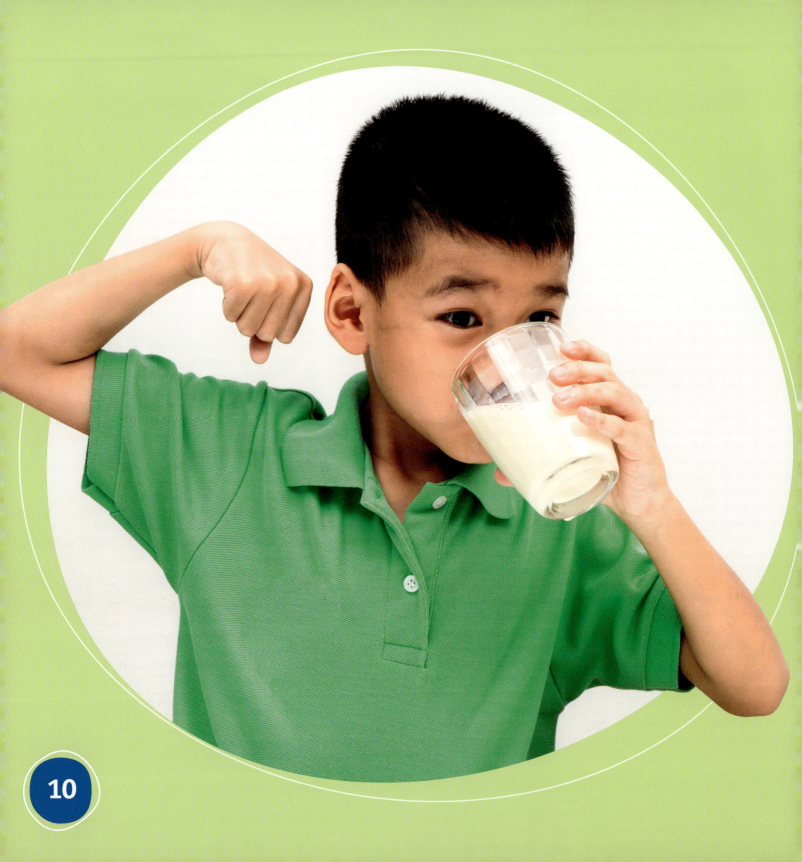

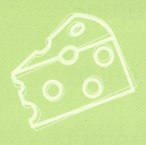
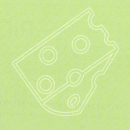

Calcium is a mineral in dairy foods.

It helps build strong bones and teeth.

Why do you think you need strong bones and teeth?

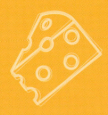

Calcium and vitamin D work together.

Vitamin D is added to milk.

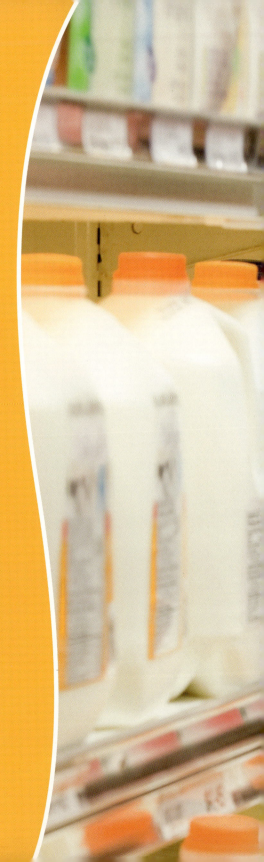

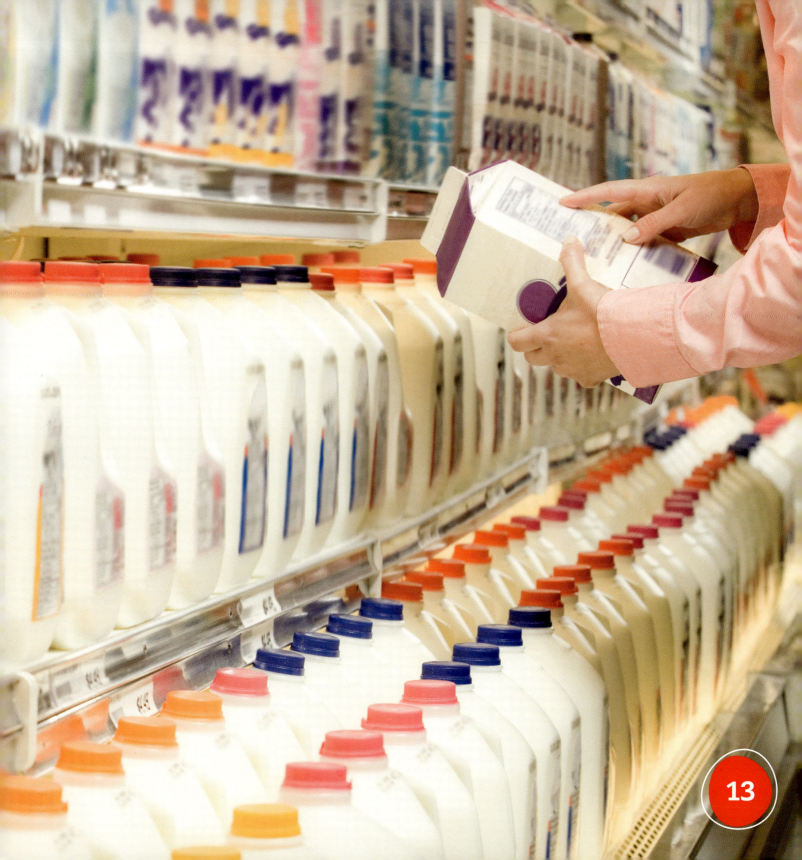

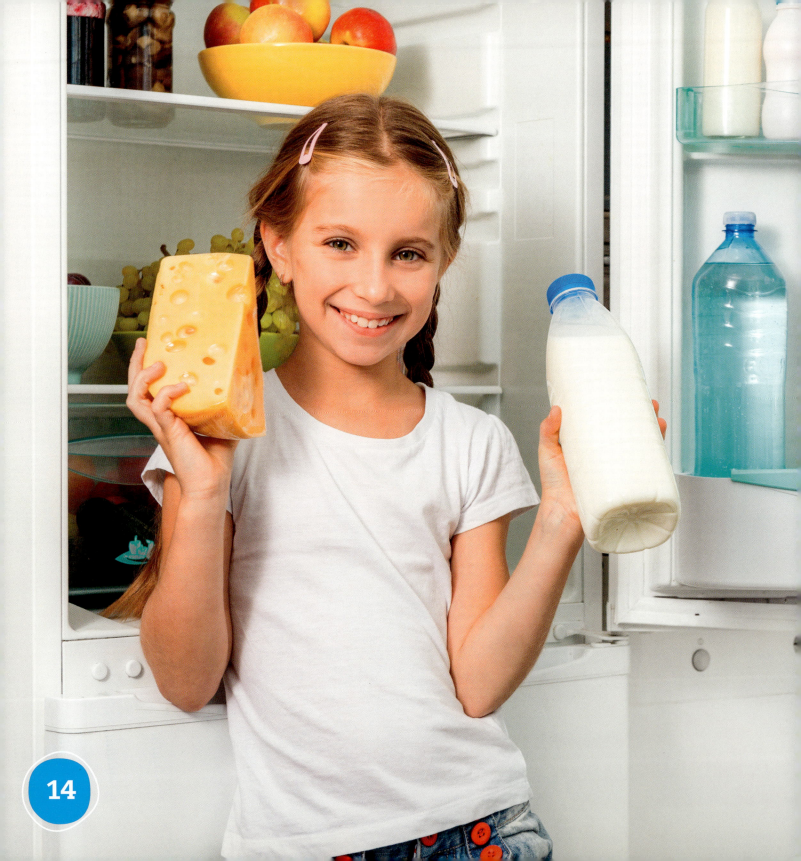

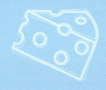

Potassium is a mineral in dairy too.

Your heart and muscles need

it to work.

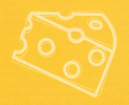

Most flavored milk has added sugar.

Flavored milk is OK sometimes.

But too much sugar is not

good for you.

Drink plain milk more often.

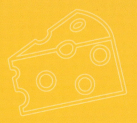

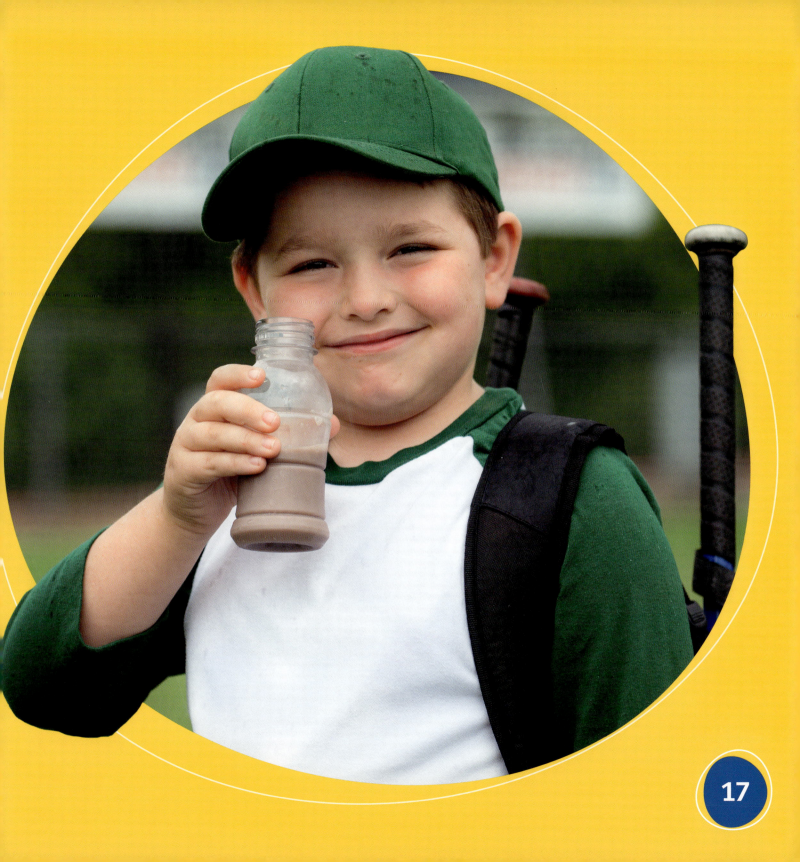

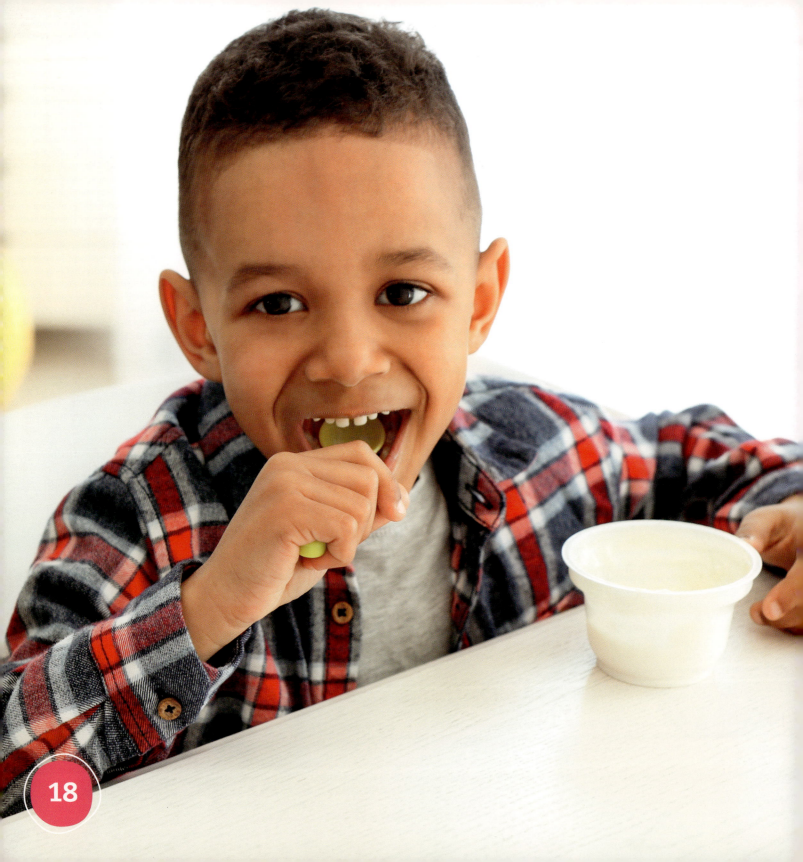

Kids need two or three servings of dairy foods daily.

Eat a cup of yogurt.

Nibble a slice of cheese.

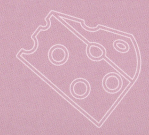

Eating dairy helps you stay healthy and strong.

What are your favorite dairy foods?

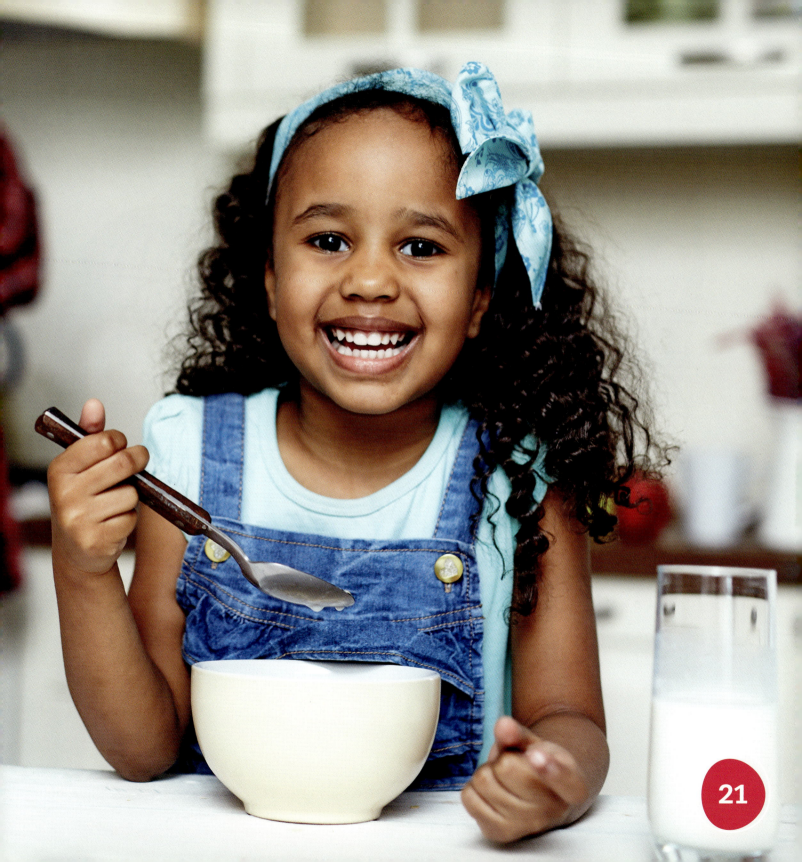

USDA MyPlate Diagram

Have milk with meals.

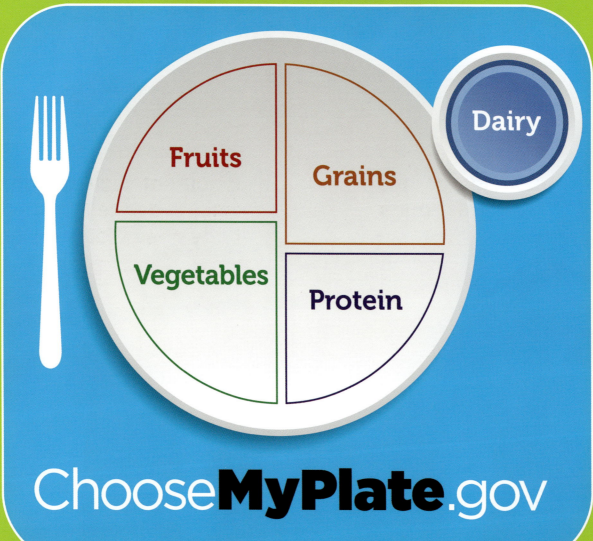

Picture Glossary

added sugar

extra sugar that is put into foods

mineral

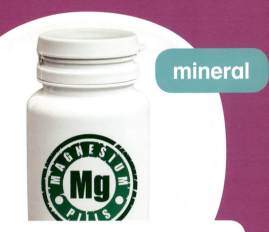

a nutrient such as iron, zinc, and others that your body needs for good health

protein

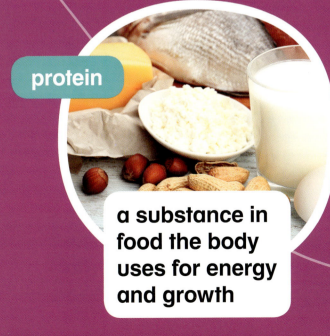

a substance in food the body uses for energy and growth

vitamin

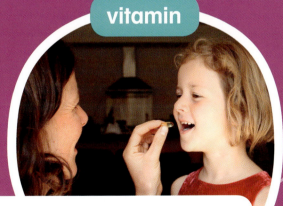

a nutrient such as vitamin A, vitamin C, and others that your body needs for good health

Read More

Black, Vanessa. *Dairy Foods.* Jump!, 2017.

Borgert-Spaniol, Megan. *Dairy Group.* Minneapolis: Bellwether Media, 2012.

Parker, Vic. *Dairy.* Irvine, CA: QEB, 2016.

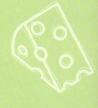
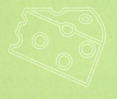

Index

added sugar, 16

calcium, 11–12

milk, 7, 12, 16

potassium, 15

protein, 8

vitamin D, 12

Photo Credits

The images in this book are used with the permission of: wavebreakmedia/Shutterstock.com, p. 5; © bitt24/Shutterstock.com, pp. 6–7, 23 (top right); © Ekaterina Markelova/Shutterstock.com, p. 9; © Oksana Kuzmina/Shutterstock.com, p. 11; © kali9/iStock.com/Shutterstock.com, p. 13; © s_oleg/Shutterstock.com, p. 14; © antoniodiaz/Shutterstock.com, p. 17; © Serhiy Kobyakov/Shutterstock.com, pp. 18, 23 (bottom right); © Pressmaster/Shutterstock.com, pp. 20–21; © US Department of Agriculture, p. 22; © kiko_jimenez/iStock.com, p. 23 (top left); © didesign021/Shutterstock.com, p. 23 (bottom left)

Front Cover: © Yulia Davidovich/Shutterstock.com